HEALTHY EATING FOR KIDS

A Parent's How-To Guide

By

Duc Vuong, M.D.

Copyright © 2016

www.UltimateGastricSleeve.com

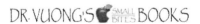

DR. VUONG'S SMALL BITES BOOKS

This book is intended for informational purposes only. This book does not offer medical advice, so nothing in it should be construed as medical advice. You should not act or rely on anything in this book or use it as a substitute for medical advice from a licensed professional. The content of this book may become outdated, especially due to the nature of the topics covered, which are constantly evolving. The information in this book is not guaranteed to be correct, complete, or timely. Certain sections of this book might have appeared in other written, audio, online, or video formats. Nothing in this book creates a doctor/patient relationship between the author and you, the reader. Although the author is a physician, he is most likely not your physician, unless he has seen you in his office as a patient. This book should not be used as a substitute to seeing your own physician.

Cover design and interior layout by Tony Loton of LOTONtech Limited.

*

Dr. Vuong's Small Bites Books provide *easily-digestible pieces of potentially life-changing information. You can find the entire series on Amazon.com.*

For every single-parent out there,

Like my father.

You inspire me every day

With your courage and relentlessness.

Introduction

*Investing in early childhood nutrition is a surefire strategy. The returns are incredibly high. – **Anne M. Mulcahy***

Good nutrition is one of the best investments we can make for our children. It deeply affects who they are today **and who they will be fifty years from now**.

As parents, we are deeply invested in the future of the upcoming generations. We want them to have every opportunity imaginable. We want them to have a good education. We want them to grow up to be happy and self sufficient. We want them to have long, healthy lives.

Good nutrition ties into all these things. A healthy lifestyle boosts the immune system, builds strong hearts and bones, and contributes to a person's overall well being. It allows the person to work at their best. They are more alert and productive. They have the fuel to get through the day and all its challenges.

Getting kids to eat healthier can be a challenge. Time and money can feel like it's in ever short supply. Some children are picky eaters. Some have food allergies. Some can not process certain things, like cow milk or gluten. Add in school, parties, and bright child-targeted marketing ads, and the whole process can feel frustrating indeed.

The good news is healthy eating is obtainable. You can start changing your child's eating habits as early as today! Contrary to popular belief, good nutrition does not need to be expensive, bland, or a daily battle of wills. Moreover, you do not need complicated recipes, exotic ingredients, or a huge budget to do it.

In this book, we are going to go over what your child's actual nutrition needs are. Then we'll go over a host of simple, practical ways to create good eating habits for every age. We will talk about when and how to introduce new foods to even the pickiest eaters. Later, we will break down the special challenges of each age. In particular, we will talk about eating outside the home.

In addition, we'll go over how to obtain healthy foods for very little. How to recognize and adjust to a food intolerance. How to meet everyone's dietary needs on a budget without extra cooking. There will even be recipes and tips that people who have never cooked can follow.

Let us get started on the foundation: **What should your child eat**?

Table of Contents

Chapter 1: Essential Childhood Nutrition

*I believe that parents need to make nutrition education a priority in their environment. – **Cat Cora (Iron Chef)***

Nutrition is more than simply filling a child's stomach. It is providing the proteins, vitamins, healthy fats and other necessary building blocks they need to grow and develop.

In their book *Generation XL,* Doctors Mercola and Lerner accurately equate our nutrition choices to building a house. Your food choices and eating habits affect every aspect of the building process **and the final result**. Cheap substitute materials and a poorly built foundation saves time and effort in the short run… but it leads to many structural problems later. As a result, it is essential to make that extra effort.

Even so, the blueprints can be hard to decipher. The sheer amount of information out there is overwhelming. It is easy to become discouraged with the many diets, studies, and programs available. One expert says give a child a food, another says to avoid it. One study says a food will lead to obesity, and another will debunk it as a myth. Even a well founded study will not fully account for the many challenges and dynamics that make a family unique.

In this chapter, we are going to go over some basic guidelines. These guidelines will build a foundation for your family**'s dietary needs**. Once you have a healthy foundation, it will be easier for you to make your own judgment calls on what works best for your family.

Dietary Needs

MyPyramid.org: There is no 'magic number' in regards to the calories and portions your child needs. It varies widely with their age, Body Mass Index (BMI), and level of activity. It does not have to be intimidating, however. The My Pyramid website is based off the current federally approved nutrition guidelines. You insert data like your child's age and activity level. Then the website interprets the results into an easy guideline of calories and recommended portion sizes. Remember, this is a 'guide,' not a prescription. It is not a substitute for more in depth knowledge or professional advice.

Healthy Fats: Children need a larger portion of healthy fats to assist in cell and brain development. In fact, throughout their developmental years it is recommended that up to a third of their calories should come from fats. **The emphasis here is 'healthy' fats**, such the kind found in avocados, nuts, whole grains and fish. Not fried foods, grease, lard, and chemically altered cooking oils.

This is especially true for the first two years of age. Allow the child to experience whole-fat milks, cheeses, and other proteins while they are in this stage of development (American Academy of Pediatrics).

Carbohydrates: Carbs have a bad reputation in the weight loss markets. This leads some people to think that carbs are 'bad' for their child. However, carbohydrates are essential in everyone's diet. They are found in fruit, vegetables, and starches that all pack fiber and essential nutrients. They provide the energy you and your child need to get through the day.

The problem comes in *quantity and quality*. We often over indulge on carbs at the expense of the other food groups. We eat more pizza, less vegetables. We eat more cereal, fewer fruits. Worse, most pre-made wheat-based carbs are 'refined'. The healthy husks are removed, and the remainder is processed into a fine white flour, which has far less nutritional value. Plus our bodies break it down too quickly, causing a roller coaster of sugar and insulin levels. **To give your child the 'slow burn' energy they need, stick with whole grain versions** (American Academy of Pediatrics).

Proteins: Proteins and amino acids are building blocks essential for the development of muscles, bones, and organs. When it comes to proteins, I advocate a pescatarian lifestyle, for nutritional purposes but also for its ease. A pescatarian is essentially a vegetarian who also eats fish and seafood. You can obtain everything you need if you are mindful about the nutrients provided. A pescatarian diet has a wide range of long term benefits. It is easier to keep 'bad' cholesterol down, and it helps you avoid other diet-related illnesses further down the line.

If the vegetarian/pescatarian lifestyle is not for your family, you can still be mindful of the type of foods you get your proteins from. Eat less beef and more eggs, beans, whole grains, and fresh fish. Keep a check on labels and know where your meats come from. Imported meats do not always follow FDA standards for health, mercury, etc. Later, I will show you how to get your kids to eat these healthier choices.

Whole Food vs Processed

Processed foods have their uses. For example, when you are traveling, a processed meal for the hotel can be very practical. The longer shelf life also makes processed canned foods good to have on hand for emergencies. And if you are in a position that you absolutely can not cook, it is handy for a meal. However, processed meals should be the exception, not the norm.

What is the problem with relying too heavily on processed foods? Processed foods are made to stay in a warehouse… then a truck… then the store shelves for weeks, months, or years before they are finally eaten. These foods are pumped full of sodium and preservatives to protect them from bacteria and decomposition. In addition, artificial colors, chemicals, sweeteners and other things are added to make the preserved food more appealing.

Whole foods are typically found around the outer rim of the grocery store. Fresh produce, fresh seafood, raw meats, and eggs are a few examples. They do not contain the sodium and additives of the pre-made foods.

Still, unless the grocery store orders from local farms, nutrients are lost in the days or weeks spent in transit. The more local your food, the more flavor and nutrition the food will have. It is surprisingly easy to find fresh ingredients right in your own community for a fraction of the price. If you are interested in eating fresh, local organic ingredients, I speak about your many practical options in my book *Eating Healthy on a Budget*.

Junk Food

Junk food is as the name implies: All calories, but few if any nutrients. Their fat, salt, and/or sugar content is very high. The proteins, vitamins, and other things the body needs are almost nonexistent. Even some proposed 'nutrition bars' and 'granola bars' can be nothing more than glorified and overpriced candy.

In general, junk foods should be cut out of the diet altogether. There are more than enough treats out there at provide for your body. For example:

- ➢ Instead of a candy bar, a fruit and nut bar provides the sweet and crunch.

- ➢ A small piece of dark cocoa provides more antioxidants for less sugar and fat than milk chocolate.

- ➢ Instead of flavored yogurt, try out smoothies from your blender or make fresh fruit and vegetable juices.

- ➢ Bake whole wheat tortilla shells into chips and make your own fresh salsa.

Hidden Junk

Some foods pose themselves as 'healthy' choices. If you look at the labels, the deception is obvious.

For example, most store bought fruit juice is not actually juice. It is made of water, fruit juice concentrates, added sugar, and preservatives. If you compare the label to a serving of the fruit, you see the juice does not have any of the nutrition of fresh fruit. You are better off spending that money on real whole fruit for your child.

Likewise, many cereals with '26 essential vitamins and minerals are primarily enriched wheat flour and sugar with vitamins artificially mixed in. Some even contain saturated fats.

Always check the labels. Pay special attention to the amount of fat and sugar in the food. Also check the ingredient list.

> ➢ Anything ending in 'ose' is a sugar. Fructose, Glucose, etc.

> ➢ Anything you can't pronounce is an artificial flavor, preservative, color or binding agent. It is important to note that some children are sensitive to one or more of these chemicals. It can cause ADD-like symptoms, indigestion, irritability and a range of other ailments.

> ➢ The ingredients are listed by quantity. For example, lets say we were looking at a banana cake. On the label it reads: Enriched White flour, Sugar, and Pureed Bananas. There is more sugar than bananas in the product, but the item is mostly flour.

Another problem with most junk foods is the 'hidden' calories. A bag of chips, a sugary cola, a couple juice pouches and a candy bar can easily **add up to a third or more of your child's daily caloric needs**. It is easy to lose track of these calories, given they are far from filling. Especially the drinks, which do not satisfy hunger and make the consumer thirsty again soon after. If the child is not active enough to burn off this overage, it is all too easy for him or her to become overweight just from these little sides and extras.

Introducing Kids to Healthier Foods

It is vital to get children into good eating habits as early as possible. The longer they are used to a habit in childhood, the more likely they are to continue the habit into adulthood. However, healthy changes can not be slammed into your lifestyle all at once. If you try to do too much, too fast, you set yourself and your child up for a difficult road.

Changes should be introduced into the child's routine gradually, especially if they already have established behavior patterns. Each change will affect everyone's habits. And the temptation to revert to the 'easier' old patterns will be strong. However, there are many easy ways to ease everyone into a healthier lifestyle.

> ➢ **Have a "New Food" Night**. Some people do not like surprises. Especially when the surprise involves a mystery meal. If you plan a specific night to try a new dish, everyone can expect to try something outside the usual menu. This allows them to mentally prepare to see something out of their comfort zone. It also breaks up the rut with a new experience. Keep the successes, and don't repeat the flops.

> ➢ **Keep It Simple**. Don't try to recreate an exotic five-star restaurant dish. There are literally thousands of good healthy dishes that any time-constrained novice could make. If they are simple and fast, they will not feel like a chore to create.

> ➢ **Make Your Own**: Have you ever paid extra for strawberry or cinnamon applesauce? Does the price of organic nut butter make you cringe? Did you know you can make these things

at home with a food processor and *no special chemicals*?

Applesauce is pureed apples. Add a peeled and cored apple with a spoonful of the ingredients you pay extra for. Puree until it is as smooth or chunky as desired. Add a few spoonfuls of water for a smoother texture.

Nut butter is a cup of unsalted nuts and a tablespoon of sunflower oil. You can experiment with the additional ingredients like dried fruit or unsweetened cocoa to make your own gourmet organic nut butter.

There are hundreds of treats that are cheaper and healthier from home. Take a day to check out your alternatives at the local library or a quick internet search. The possibilities are endless.

Before Changing a Child's Diet

➤ **Know Their Threshold.** Children love to explore and try new things. However, they also want to feel safe within an ordained set of boundaries. When the balance is tipped, they become resistant and the battle commences. If you are mindful about how much change your child can tolerate, you can introduce new things at a pace they will be comfortable with. This will greatly reduce mealtime warfare.

➤ **Consult An Expert.** A pediatrician or child nutritionist can give you valuable insight regarding your child's individual dietary needs. They can give you ideas on what to expect, and any challenges you may face. They can also provide information you need to make the new diet effective.

➤ **Small, Simple Steps**. It's tempting to just jump in and try to do it all at once. This is a quick path to frustration and resistance. Start off with small steps to get everyone used to the changes first. For example, swapping from whole milk to 2%, then skim or fat-free. If you are swapping to almond milk, mix cow milk with a dose of almond milk. Increase the ratio of almond milk over time until they are drinking it exclusively.

Small steps are less overwhelming and easier to maintain than a sudden shift.

> ➢ **Never Join A Fad**. The latest new miracle diet will sound wonderful. However, most 'revolutionary' eating plans are incredibly flawed. Case in point was the Atkin's For Kids diet, where parents were encouraged to feed children high amounts of protein while restricting carbs to almost nothing. It was 'the' perfect diet that made pediatricians cringe. As we discussed earlier, carbohydrates are in your fruits and vegetables and are necessary for energy. Do your research before subscribing to any plan.

> ➢ **Be Mindful**. When your child is resistant to trying a new food, try to identify the source. A child's vocabulary and ability to self-diagnose are limited. They speak in colorful if vague descriptions like "yucky" and "icky." They have trouble articulating that some fruits make them light headed and irritable. They do not know that the rosemary in the dinner is what made their tummy hurt in the middle of the night. They do not know that the bad feeling they get after eating the new pasta dish is a gluten allergy. You will need to watch for patterns and context to fill in these blanks.

> ➢ **Everyone Follows The Same Rules**. Double standards will only serve to confuse the message. The child may see their new diet as unfair and resent their available food choices. To keep the focus on a healthy lifestyle, everyone in the

household should practice the same rules. If a child can only have healthy snacks, then teens and grownups must act as role models. If a child can not have a sugary drink, do not buy a soda for yourself.

➢ **Body Image**. Body image is very important to children, especially tweens and teenagers. Society pushes very unhealthy images in all forms of media. The more social their everyday life becomes, the more sensitive they can learn to be to their image. It is easy for a child to assume the new menu of healthy food is because they are 'fat.'

Make sure they understand that the new diet has nothing to do with being skinny or physically attractive. It is about good health and energy. Also emphasize this is a 'diet' as in a good lifelong eating habit, not the 'lose weight' diets they see on TV.

There are hosts of simple ways to make healthy choices when you change up the menu. If you are mindful, you will even be able to make the transition fun and painless for you and your child.

It does not need to stop there. You can also empower yourself to keep your child eating healthy no matter where they are. Let's go over ways to keep your child eating healthy in any situation.

Chapter 2: Taking Control

If you keep good food in your fridge,
*You will eat good food. – **Errick McAdams***

Good health boils down to making healthy foods available, and limiting the rest. You are a powerful force in your child's life. You are their guide and their advocate in a world that makes unhealthy choices far too convenient.

Even if you have never cooked a meal in your life, you can start to take control of your family's eating habits today.

Moderation

Keep in mind, life is not perfect. You will go to a game where food is limited to soda and greasy meats. They will attend sleepovers where the main meal might be pizza rolls and a 2 pound bag of M&M's. You will go to an event that avoids whole foods like the plague. Do not panic.

Singular events like these will not ruin your child for life. Make them an interesting exception rather than the norm. Focus on avoiding foods that might trigger their allergies. Make the best decisions you can, and go with the flow on the rest.

In fact, I encourage small indulgences. A small piece of chocolate now and then keeps you from craving the treat as a 'forbidden fruit.' The trick is to be mindful of how much and how often you indulge. If you completely forbid a food, the healthier lifestyle will start to feel like a restriction. It makes the banned foods more desirable.

Home

The home is your territory and primary battleground. This is the one place you have complete control over the meals served. You control what is in the fridge and pantry. You choose what snacks to keep on hand.

With that in mind, how do so many junk foods and processed meals end up in our territory? In short: Price and Convenience. A cheap and fast microwave dinner has a lot of appeal when you are in a hurry and on a budget.

While these foods are convenient, they are also shoddy building materials. They only serve to cut corners. Long term they reduce the quality of the body they build.

This does not mean fresh, healthy food has to be expensive or time consuming. There are lots of ways to get the quality at a lower price.

> **You Can Make Anything.** Vegetable soup, chicken and rice, fish sticks... Everything on the shelf and in the freezer aisle can be made fresh from scratch, with better ingredients, and no preservatives or artificial colors. **This is the best option because you know exactly what is in your child's food.**

> **Make Extra.** You do not need to scrub pots and pans every night. Pick a day to make meals in bulk, then portion them into containers you can store and rewarm later in the week. Make extra portions for work and school lunches, or busy nights. Some super planners even do all their cooking once a month!

> **Extra portions are also handy for school lunches or when you host a last minute sleepover**. You can provide a real meal to the group with no extra work involved.

> **Trade Off**. Do you make great eggplant lasagna? Double up and trade the dish with a friend or neighbor for one of their

healthy recipes. This is a great way to get something new on the table that you did not cook yourself.

➤ **Invest In A Slow Cooker**. A slow cooker is the best friend of any busy, healthy lifestyle. You place the ingredients in the pot and set the time. It cooks while you work, clean, pick up children, and other life events. It is not limited to roasts and casseroles like older models. There are recipes for various specialty foods like gluten free vegetarian pizza and fresh bread online.

➤ **Eat Slowly**. Encourage everyone at the dinner table to slow down and eat slowly. It takes around 15 minutes for your stomach to tell the brain that it is full. When we race through our meals we tend to over eat. Instead of forks and spoons, try eating with chopsticks. This will definitely slow down your meal, while providing you with more than a few memorable   laughs.

Eating slowly allows everyone to enjoy the taste and experience of the food. You also give yourself a chance to 'tire' of the taste, so you are less likely to go back for seconds and thirds.

This is especially helpful with junk foods. When indulging, your child will need less to be satisfied... they might not even like the food when they actually slow down enough to taste it!

➤ **Try Out Vegetarian Recipes**. Even those who do not embrace a full vegetarian lifestyle can benefit from trying meatless alternatives. Start off with favorite foods like pizza and spaghetti. Try black beans instead of ground beef. See if your family likes soy or tofu recipes. Meat tends to be the most expensive ingredient in a dish. Cutting meat reduces the fat content, and the vegetables add in vitamins, fiber, and nutrients.

➢ **Add A Protein To Salad**. Proteins help make a salad more interesting and satisfying. Try shredded chicken or grilled shrimp. Add in nuts for a pleasant crunch. Add beans instead of a calorie filled dressing. Mix in Tuna with a light Italian dressing instead of mayonnaise.

➢ **Shop Local**. Get acquainted with the local markets, like the butcher and fishmonger. Know the dates and locations of the Farmer's Market during the growing season. Keep an eye out on local community sites like Bookoo and Craigslist for people selling or giving away surplus produce or eggs. The more you look, the more options for affordable, fresh and healthy foods you will find.

➢ **Sales Circulars**: In my earlier book, *Eating Healthy on a Budget*, I explained the importance of using sales and circulars to plan your shopping trips. You see all their best sales before you ever step out the door. You know when the sale is, which store has the best value, what to stock up in bulk on. In addition, you eventually start to identify patterns in the sales.

➢ **Go Local**: Get to know your local food sources. The butcher can custom cut your meat, or make ground hamburger without the filler and extra fat. You can even ask them to slice, dice and grind leaner cuts of meat for you at no additional cost. Often, the butcher and fishmongers have monthly specials or package deals as well, saving you money on fresh food than was not frozen in a warehouse for weeks.

> **Farmer's Market**: During the growing season, you can frequent your local farmer's market for fresh produce, homemade cheeses, local honey, and other goods. It is much fresher than the produce you find at the supermarket, which usually spends weeks to months on trucks and in warehouses before it hits the produce aisle.

> **Watch Labels**. If cooking is not for you, you can still keep an eye on the nutrition labels. Aim for pre-made foods with five or fewer ingredients, steamable bags, and all natural ingredients. While it is not as cost effective as cooking for yourself, you will still improve your child's meals considerably.

Feeding Multiple children

> **Same Food, Different Portions**. Everyone eats the same thing, but the portions are served according to individual needs. Some people fall into the trap of trying to make a special dish for each person at the table.

For example, instead of making a gluten-free pancake for one child and regular whole grain pancakes for everyone else you can buy a healthy gluten free version in bulk. Then make enough gluten free pancakes for the whole family. You'll find the price comparable to making the two versions separately. However, the time and effort is reduced.

> **Buy Staples In Bulk**: Buy the staples in large bulk. There are many staples like brown rice, wheat noodles, oats, beans, lentils, and quinoa that can be used for a multitude of dishes. Add a handful to soup stock with some vegetables. Try out different spices in a bake or casserole.

> **Bulk Stores**. Stores like Costco, Smart and Final, and Sam's Club sell food in large bulk for a significant discount off the unit price. In fact, many small businesses, clubs, and charity events use these stores to shop when they need less than a pallet of a product.

Thrifty Tip: Don't need 5 dozen eggs for $3.00? Don't want to buy 10 of an item to get the massive discount? Pair up with one or more other families. Split the cost and the products!

Babysitters and Relatives

There are times when someone else will affect your child's eating habits. Very few babysitters want the responsibility or liability of firing up the oven. In fact, in our modern convenient culture, some have never even cooked a day in their lives.

> **Have Something Prepared**. If your child will be in another's care at mealtime, prepare a meal they can share together. The caretaker will appreciate it, and be less compelled to feed them a junk food.

> **Don't Keep It In The House**. If there is no junk food in the house, the caretaker can not feed it to your child. Keep some baby carrots and dipping sauce or pre-sliced fruit on hand for handy snacks. If they are going to the caretaker's home, be sure to let them know ahead of time if you plan to send meals or snacks.

> **Choose Your Battles**. When dealing with relatives, it is inevitable that some will want to indulge your child. Some see sweets and junk foods as having fun or 'living a little.' Sweet foods are also sometimes seen as an easy way to bond and show affection.

Don't be the bouncer at the gate. Instead, find comfortable boundaries you can both agree with. For example, you could agree that they give the child a snack sized candy instead of a full sized bar. You could make Nana the exclusive source of their favorite fruit treat. You can also agree on other ways to indulge a child. For example, they could take the child to a skating rink, watch a treasured movie together, or share their favorite hobby.

> ➤ **Keep A List**. Make sure to write down mealtimes, snacks, and allergies for the caretaker. That way they will have a clear vision of what is expected of them. **You can find an example list in Appendix 2 of this book.**

> ➤ **Keep Active:** When your child does eat junk food, follow up with a brief physical activity. If they ran and played in the time frame, don't sweat it. They already got the exercise. Even if they are very active, don't let it be an excuse to overindulge on foods with no nutrition to them.

These are just a few ways you can reclaim control when others are involved. With practice, quick solutions and reasonable compromises will become second nature.

Dining Out

If you do dine out, you can still keep your family from eating two thousand calories or more in one sitting. Here are a few practical tips:

> ➤ **Cut Back On Fast Food**. You pay a price for the saved time and convenience. Namely in high calories, sodium, and fats. Research places that serve fresh foods. There are often many hidden 'mom and pop' family restaurants that serve fresh home-style cooking. There is also a rise in diners and cafes specifically geared to healthy eating.

➢ **Avoid Buffets**. Buffets are made to feed a mass of people quickly. This is not the same as serving fresh and nutritious foods. In addition, the temptation to overeat from the wide selection is high.

➢ **Go a La Carte Or Substitute**. When ordering, avoid the standard fries and soda combo. Either pick up the main items you came in for. You can also see if they will substitute the sides for water and a healthier side item like a salad, steamed vegetables, or some fruit.

➢ **Split Plates.** Before ordering, look at their portion sizes. Most restaurants serve oversized servings. Split these jumbo plates into smaller portions to share instead of a kid's meal.

➢ **Go Lean:** Opt for grilled instead of fried. Stick to leaner meats like chicken and fish. Try out the bean and vegetarian alternatives on the menu, if available. Black bean burgers are very tasty!

➢ **Skip The Bread**. While you wait for your food, a restaurant often offers complimentary bread with a rich butter to flavor it. By the time the nutritious food arrives your child is already full. Instead, ask about a less filling substitute or skip the filler altogether.

➢ **Skip The Dessert**. Like the bread, most desserts are fillers that do not have a nutritional value. It takes 15 minutes for our brains to process that we are full. We do not usually have that much time to decide in a restaurant. Instead, wait until you get home. If your child still craves something sweet by then, you will at least have a wide variety of healthy options like yogurt, some applesauce or a small fruit smoothie. Even if you let them indulge in a chocolate or small candy, you have more control over portions at home than on a restaurant menu.

Holidays and Special Events

The holidays can be a more difficult time to keep a child on a healthy routine. You want them to have all the fun and life experiences but not the overflow of junk foods that accompany it.

Sweet treats were originally *a treat*. Sugar and candy was not readily available like it is today. There were no vending machines and checkout aisle candy bars. The cakes and pies and candies were a gift to get excited about. They were only bought or made on special occasions. A fresh pie, a sweet cake, or a few candies were something to get excited about!

Nowadays sugar is awarded in great excess. The holiday treat is no longer necessarily a rare indulgence. It has become an annual avalanche of sugar and fats. At the same time, they are so ingrained into our holiday traditions that it can feel difficult to cut them out altogether.

There are lots of great ways to handle this dilemma without policing your child through the holidays. For example:

- ➤ **Halloween**: Let them dress up and go trick or treating. Then let them keep a set portion. Offer to buy the rest at an agreed upon price. You can then dispose of the excess.

  - ◦ **Cool Tip**: Check with halloweencandybuyback.com for places in your local area. These places purchase candy to get them off the streets. Then they send the candies in care packages to troops overseas!

- ➤ **Thanksgiving**: Indulge a little, but only go for one helping and one small dessert. Serve the dessert on a small, interesting plate to make it more appealing. Follow up with games that encourage running and exercise to let kids burn off extra calories. This is also great for parties, reunions, and weddings.

➢ **Christmas**: Fewer candy canes, more hot apple cider and orange slices. Fewer video game consoles. More bikes, skateboards, climbing ropes, Frisbees and other things that encourage kids to be active. If you live in tight spaces, consider doorway swing-sets, light-foam balls that bounce harmlessly off breakables, and mini trampolines if space allows.

Mix parties with physical activity like walks to see the holiday lights or an after party romp through the park. Don't eat sweets at EVERY party. Save it for the best desserts.

➢ **Easter.** Put a few small favorite candies in their basket. Check out a dollar store to fill in the rest with inflatable toys, jump ropes, art supplies, and other fun stuff to keep their minds and bodies active. Fill the eggs with stickers of favorite characters, small novelties, pocket change, and low sugar treats.

➢ **Vacations.** Treat vacations like extended parties. Enjoy but try not to overindulge. Keep the majority of your food choices on track. Split large portions. Make sure you have some physical activities on the itinerary.

With a little ingenuity, you can keep the holidays from getting out of hand. This gets even easier when you know exactly what your child needs and when.

Chapter 3: Infants and Toddlers

Some people care too much. I think it is called Love. – A.A Milne

This stage of development is probably the easiest to change. The infant or toddler is still getting used to eating in general. Their tastes are going to constantly change and evolve. They are also at an age where they put everything in their mouths. They will be more open to exploring their world with new tastes and experiences.

Starting Solids:

According to registered dietician Karen Ansel, a baby will let you know when they are ready to start solid foods. You should start looking for signs when they can sit upright with support and hold their own head steady. They will show interest in what you are eating, and the baby will lean forward and open his or her mouth when food is offered.

Keep in mind that the baby is primarily exploring the concept of eating. It will not replace formula in the near future. In fact, a baby just starting out on solids will only eat a spoonful or two. **When this happens, it is important not to force it.** They will eat larger quantities as they develop and gain practice (Altman et al).

When introducing a baby to new foods, it is best to start with one ingredient at a time. Watch them for 3 to 5 days as you feed them for signs of a food allergy or intolerance. By limiting the experience, you can quickly pinpoint when a food is wrong for the baby. **See Appendix 1 for a handy worksheet to copy and record your progress** for you and your pediatrician.

Make Your Own Baby Food

Making baby food at home is very simple and economical. You just need a good food processor. You can make meals for the rest of the family, then puree baby's portion with a little water, breast milk or formula. No salt or spices. Freeze any extra in ice trays and then store away for later.

This has a large range of benefits. First, you know for a fact what your baby is eating. You blended it yourself. Second, the baby food is fresh! **You might be surprised that some of those jars in the baby food aisle are older than the baby eating them (Alter et al)!** That can be a real eye opener when it comes to how preservatives affect our food. You know for a fact there is no sugar, sodium, or anything artificial in the food. It is only pureed carrots, cooked squash, or whatever is on the baby's menu for the day.

Finally, it is very economical. If the family is having carrots as a side dish, you set aside a few spoonfuls of cooked carrots to process into baby food. You are not paying out extra grocery money. You are not hoarding boxes of empty glass jars in the back storage. You are simply freezing the excess to thaw for another day.

When to Introduce Them to Foods

> **Soft Fruits:** Soft fruits that can be mashed with a fork can be introduced once the baby is ready to start eating. Avocados and bananas are good places to start. They are very high in fiber and potassium, among other nutrients. Peel and process soft fruits in a food processor with enough water, breast milk or formula to make it very smooth and almost fluid. After about eight weeks, you can fork mash and offer your infant small bites.

> **Eggs**. A baby can start eating eggs as early as six months. It is a handy source of proteins and healthy fats. Cook the egg without butter, then puree it with a little breast milk or formula to make it easier to chew and swallow. You can make extra in the morning along with everyone's meal.

> ➢ **Thrifty Extra**: Eggs reheat fast. You can make a school week's worth of eggs in bulk for the whole family to ensure everyone (including baby) gets a fast and easy protein boost in the mornings.

> ➢ **Cow Milk**. For the first year, baby should not drink cow milk. The still-developing digestive system is not ready to process the complex proteins, and it could lead to intolerance later. However, a baby can eat small amounts of yogurt and cheese by six months (Altman).

> ➢ **Yogurt**: Babies can have yogurt by around six months. The best is a no fake color option with live cultures. These will help develop a healthy digestive and immune system (Altman)

> ➢ **Honey**. A baby should not be introduced to honey in the first year. Their immune and digestive systems are not equipped to deal with any amount of botulism that might be present. It is potentially fatal, especially if the toxic spores start growing in baby's undeveloped intestines (Mayo clinic).

Baby Language

While your infant and toddler do not have a working vocabulary language yet, they have ways to communicate. For example, if your baby turns away from food, or they back away from the spoon, they had enough. If they only ate a few bites it is alright. They still mostly depend on milk or formula in the early stages. See a pediatrician's advice if you suspect they are refusing food in general.

If they cry or get fussy soon after eating certain foods, they may have gas or an intolerance to an ingredient. **Keep the eating journal in appendix 1 to watch for patterns.** Check with your pediatrician if necessary.

Toddlers:

Toddlers start to develop eating skills quickly after they move past purees. By age one, they can practice holding a spoon while you feed them. By age two they are able to self-feed bite-sized portions, and they show greater interest in choosing their food.

> ➢ **More Patience.** In this stage, children learn the word 'no.' They may even refuse food for the simple fact that they can. You may need to introduce a new 'icky' food many times over the course of weeks or months before they finally try their first bite.

> ➢ **Their Tastes Change**: As they develop their palette, the child will suddenly reject favorite foods. They might even want vast quantities of foods they avoided in the past. **This is normal.** Try to take it in good stride if they decide they don't like blueberries the day after you bought several containers worth. Vacuum seal and freeze these foods in hopes that they remember these lost loves in the near future. Most foods will last for a year or more in this way.

> ➢ **Choices**: Do not become a short order cook. However, by age 2 they become more opinionated about their meals. Let them make small decisions like which bowl they will use, or what fruit they want on their yogurt. This will give them practice in making choices within healthy boundaries.

> ➢ **Food Intake**: The American Academy of Pediatrics recommends that children get about 40 calories a day for every inch of height. You can print out a custom serving chart for your child at MyPyramid.org.

> ➢ **Limit Screen Time**. All tech off at mealtime. This will help your child enjoy their food and identify when they are full. Also, some children are growing up without a clue how to

deal with the world without a screen. Human face-to-face time and fewer distractions will help them cope with the world as they get older. Use the time to teach them good table manners and conversation, or hear what they are thinking about. Children's imaginations can be amazing entertainment at the dinner table.

➤ **Always Cut It For Them**. Though they can eat the same foods, choking hazards are still a real possibility. Make sure everything is cut into small pieces. Starting out, no bigger than a Cheerio. As they get older and more experienced, move up to bite-sized pieces.

➤ **Practice Makes Perfect.** They can practice spearing and spooning foods with age appropriate child dinnerware. Make sure the tips have rounded edges and they are labeled BPH free.

➤ **Keep Introducing New Things**. Give your child something familiar that you know they will eat, and then a couple of spoonfuls of something new on the side. Continue the three-day observation on one new ingredient at a time to identify potential food allergies.

➤ **Prepackaged Toddler Meals**. Like most shelf foods, the majority of prepackaged toddler meals and snacks are loaded with sodium and preservatives to extend their shelf life. It is better to make your own at home. However, these prepackaged meals are still handy for long travel, hotel stays and vacations.

➤ **Fewer "Kid" Foods**. The enticing dinosaur shapes, colorful cereal mascots, and special pastas are all marketed toward children. However, when you inspect the label, these foods are not made with child-nutrition in mind. Have them eat the same foods as everyone else at the dinner table.

These are just a few examples of great ways to let a child explore the world of healthy foods. It will take practice to achieve healthy boundaries, but it will be well worth it when your child reaches school age.

Chapter 4: Preschool and Kindergarten

A child's body needs nutrition. Not just food. – **Julie Webb Kelley**

Preschool is a challenging stage for your child's health. They are spending more time in another person's care. He or she is exposed to the standards of the school and their peers. They eat at the times the school allots to them, and they have to eat foods the school allows.

In addition, your child is starting to be more active in the community. There are clubs, sports and recitals. Party invitations start to become more common. You have more errands and events to run to. Some days will feel like an absolute whirlwind of activity.

This does not mean you can not continue to provide your child a healthy lifestyle. There are lots of ways to maintain your child's throughout the school year.

School

➤ **Check The School**: Examine the school's nutritional environment. Look over their menus, ask what companies supply the ingredients and check them out. Find out how to get regular updates about their weekly menu. Don't forget to check out their vending machines and concession stands if applicable. Knowledge will help you plan out when your child should bring their own lunch (Altman).

➤ **Discuss Good Choices**: Discuss good health choices with your child so they have the ability to make good choices. There will be days that they swap their yogurt for someone's junk food. However, reminding them about good foods can help them make better choices.

➢ **Purchase An Insulated Thermos And Lunch Sack**. The well made ones are pricier, but they will keep foods the right temperature until lunchtime. If you need a quick fix, slip a reusable hot/cold pack in their lunch box in the morning.

Home

➢ **Limit Screen Time**: Sitting around for long periods is not good for them. In addition, the commercials on their favorite shows are specially geared to tantalize them. They are tested and specially made to make children want and desire sweets and junk foods. In addition, most cartoons depict their heroes drinking sodas and eating burgers, nachos or pizza.

➢ **All Tech Off At Mealtime**: This includes the television. Make it a time to find out about school, their new favorite games, and just communicate. This gives them the necessary interaction skills to socialize with people later down the road.

➢ **Prep Ahead:** You can save yourself time if you plan meals in advance. Make foods over the weekend to rewarm during the busy school week. Eggs keep will in the freezer; you can rewarm them for a fast protein boost for breakfast. Dry whole grain cereal can be poured into a bowl and left in the fridge. Leftovers can be poured into individual containers for lunches. Double batch dinner recipes and freeze half for another night.

➢ **Do Not Let Weekends Slip**: After a busy week, it can be tempting to fall back on cheap and fast fixes and let them spend the day glued to screens. However, this loss of structure is not good for either of you. Keep a routine of structured mealtimes and physical activity.

- ○ **Super Tip:** If you stored away extra leftovers through the week, then you will have several meals ready to rewarm and serve. This also saves you the cost of a whole meal!

- ➤ **Keep Water And Granola In Vehicle**: Water and granola keep well in various temperatures. Keep them in the trunk or a small container. That way, if you and your child get hungry on the go, you have a snack handy. If you buy premade granola or cereal bars, make sure to read the labels. Most of the popular ones are more sugar than granola.

- ➤ **Avoid "Fillers" For Snacks**. Breads and crackers can fill up a small stomach before the more nutritious mealtime. Stick with a few baby carrots, some apple slices, or other healthy snacks that leave room for mealtime.

Helping In The Kitchen

You can further reinforce your child's awareness of healthy choices by letting them help you around the kitchen. This will help develop an independent and healthy lifestyle later in life.

- ➤ **Lead By Example.** Everything your child learns about food will come from *what you show, not what you say*. Eat the foods you want them to eat. Cut back on soda and snacking. Eat sweets in moderation. Whatever your rules are, live by them. It will benefit you both if you are your child's role model in healthy eating.

- ➤ **Reorganize**. Put their bowls, plates, and cups in a lower cabinet so that they can choose their own. Let them set their place at the table.

➢ **Let Them Help**. Let them do simple tasks for mealtime like shredding lettuce, whisking eggs, skewering fruit onto kabobs, or smashing nuts in a bag (Altman). This will make healthy cooking less foreign and intimidating later.

➢ **Stock Up**. Keep fruit and easy to snack on vegetables on hand. These make a good snack between meals and additions to a lunch box. Keep air-pop popcorn, dried fruit and pretzels on hand in place of chips.

Rewards

Comfort eating often comes from when food was used as a reward or a consolation. This can lead to eating problems later in life, especially when they start dealing with stress, testing, and peer pressure later in life. Find rewards and comforts that do not involve food. There are plenty of ways to indulge or reward a child without adding a single extra calorie.

➢ **Cater To Their Interests**. If they like bugs, go out bug catching together. If they like princesses, find some crafting ideas on Pinterest to make them some accessories. If they like puzzles, print out one from PBSkids.org. Each child is different. If you keep yourself aware of their interests, you can find a multitude of great ideas.

➢ **Family Time**. Sometimes your undivided attention is all they could ever need or want. Read a book together. Play a board game. Solve a puzzle. Talk about something they like with no outside interruptions.

➢ **Free Entertainment**: Libraries are not just books anymore. You can also find CDs and movies. Most active libraries also have several children's programs and clubs throughout the week! Depending on your area, you may even find a children's book club or a weekly science experiment.

➤ **Free Entertainment**: A trip to the park or a walking trail can provide great outdoor entertainment. You could also pitch a tent on the patio or build a blanket fort in the living room.

➤ **Points.** Let them build up points for good grades and behavior. These points could be redeemed toward a day at the zoo, a small art/science kit, a puzzle book, or other enriching reward. There are also some great creative and educational apps they could enjoy during their limited screen time instead of cartoons.

While your child is not under your constant vigil, you can still keep them full of healthy, nutritious foods with some extra effort and planning. Preschool and Kindergarten are a great time to hammer out the basics. As they get older, things start to get more challenging.

Chapter 5: Grade School

Teaching kids how to feed themselves and how to live in a community responsibly is the center of an education. – Alice Waters

As children get older, they get busier, and unhealthy foods start to become more accessible. They have more access to vending machines through their school day. After-school games are celebrated at fast food locations. They spend more time hanging out with friends, participating in parties, and some start attending sleepovers.

In addition, they will take keen interest in what their friends are doing. The games they play. The shows they watch. The kind of online game systems their friends hang out on. The food they eat. The older they get, the more these observations will shape their behavior as they 'fit in' with their friends.

In addition, each year is a brand new attempt to achieve work-life balance. You may have to balance work and home on top of the homework, events, and activities.

Check Out School

Before the school year begins, know everything about your school's nutritional standards. What do they serve for lunch? Where can you attain a copy of their menu? What is in their vending machines or concession stand? How do they deal with food allergies?

Chances are you will need to pack some or all of your child's lunches. This is easy to do if you store away the leftovers or extra batches in individual containers. Just heat it in the morning and pack it in a well insulated lunch container.

> ➤ **Frozen Smoothie**. If the school allows, you can freeze a fruit smoothie over night. By the time it thaws, it will be ready to drink for a lunch supplement.

➤ **Temperature Control**. If their food is lukewarm by the time lunch arrives, insert a reusable hot or cold pack into their lunch bags in the morning to keep the correct temperature longer. If they are responsible with their lunch bags, upgrade to a better insulated one.

➤ **Utensils**. Pack disposable utensils in their bags. If they are brought home, wash and reuse.

➤ **Add A Protein**. When packing lunches and snacks, add a protein to make it more satisfying. For example, chopped fruit and some yogurt, celery and homemade peanut butter, or a salad with quinoa.

➤ **Boiled Eggs**. You can peel and soak a hard-boiled egg in sweet vinegar or beet juice to add flavor without salt. Make sure the flavorings have low or no sodium added. They can eat it as-is or add it to a salad.

➤ **Practice Responses**. A child who brings quinoa and smoked salmon to school is bound to have questions and comments directed at them sooner or later. If they seem uncomfortable with bringing a food to school, discuss the concern and help them come up with responses to their peers.

Note: Give a "concern time" and consideration. Even if the problem seems 'silly' from an adult standpoint, it is very real and very big to a child. They have fewer life experiences for context. In addition, the children teasing them do not have that life context either. As a result, their problem with your child's food choices is a lot more significant in their minds. Do not dismiss a child's concerns too quickly.

Kitchen

Too many modern children lack even rudimentary cooking skills when they leave the nest. In fact, cooking might even feel intimidating. As a result, they rely almost exclusively on processed foods and restaurants for nourishment. It is important to get your kids acquainted with cooking as early as possible. My daughter, Kizzie, started cooking with me around the age of 4. She loved spinning the salad spinner and rolling lemons. By age 5, she was peeling vegetables and softening onions on the stove top.

> ➤ **You Do Not Need To Be A Chef**. It's okay if you've never cooked in your life. Learning together can be a great bonding experience for you both. You'll both benefit by learning and sharing new life skills.

> ➤ **Let Them Help**. Grade school age children can help shred lettuce, peel and mash potatoes, peel eggs, etc. Each child matures differently. Use your best judgment on when they are ready to bake, use a blender, chop vegetables, make their own whole wheat pancakes, etc.

> ➤ **Be Patient.** They will not do it exactly the way you would do it. They might miss a few places on the carrot. They might not be as sanitary as you'd like. They might lose interest and run off. They also might get burned or cut. Use these as teaching points.

> ➤ **Let Them Help Shop**. Give them the list and put them in charge of checking off the found items. Let them check prices and labels for specific clues (Find a granola bar with whole oats as the first ingredient or Find the best price on fresh tomatoes.) Let them weigh out the produce then calculate the cost of it. These small steps will help them do their own shopping later in life, as well as be cognizant of spending.

Rewards

Their world grows gradually more complicated with each school year. It is all too tempting to reward or console a child with a snack or comfort food. This sets them up for 'comfort eating' later in life. Luckily, there are hundreds of ways to replace food as an indulgence. Here are a few examples to get you started.

- ➤ **Age Appropriate Places To Visit**. When they do well, go out someplace they would enjoy. Visit a zoo or aquarium. Take a free experimental class at the library. Go to a pool or a park.

- ➤ **Giant Rolls Of Paper**. You can purchase a roll of paper from a hobby shop, or get the end roll from some printing shops for a decent price. Create an art wall or let them redecorate the inside of their door.

- ➤ **Points**. Do they want to see a movie coming out soon, or want to try a karate class? Let them accumulate points for good grade, behavior, chores, etc. When they have enough points, they earn a set reward.

- ➤ **Get Out Of Chore Free Card**. On a special occasion, give them a card that they can redeem to avoid a chore for a day. Make sure the rules for redeeming are clear, such as "You can not use it to avoid cleaning your room before the weekend." or "The chore must be claimed before breakfast is over."

Field Trips and Events

- ➤ **Stock Up**. Keep 'quick to cook' meals handy in the freezer for band and sports meets. That way you can warm their meals while everyone gets ready for school, or right before you drop it off for an evening game.

➤ **Hands On Foods.** On event days, prepare foods that can be eaten with one hand. While the group should have picnic tables handy, there is always a possibility they will eat picnic style or on the bus. Avoid messy foods that could spill or splatter all over in an awkward handhold.

➤ **Eating Out**. If kids are going to eat at a restaurant, find out if bringing meals is an option. Briefly remind your child about the healthier choices they can make, and remind their chaperones of any food allergies or health concerns.

➤ **Sandwiches**. Keep pickles, tomatoes and other wet ingredients to the side in small container. Use whole grain or seed bread instead of white bread. Choose healthier meats other than deli meats, like roasted chicken. Go light or skip condiments being a spoonful can pack significant calories.

➤ **Pack Water**. Gatorade, sodas, and juice pouches are loaded with sodium, sugar and preservatives. Keep kids away from energy drinks and shots. There is far more sugar and caffeine in them than their bodies should be exposed to. Make them fresh protein and vitamin fortified smoothies and shakes instead.

Tweens and Eating Problems

Tweens are in that awkward stage between childhood and the teenage years. They are growing ever more sensitive to their social network and the opinions of their peers. Beloved interests and hobbies will come and go practically overnight. Fads and new games or trends will be pursued like it is a matter of life and death. In this turmoil, their opinion on food will also change with feedback from their peers.

It is also a very vulnerable time. Most tweens, especially young girls, crave the approval and attention of their peers. Bullying, self-esteem issues, and eating disorders are all very real threats to your child's physical and psychological well being.

> **Keep In Touch**. Listen to what your child is interested in, even if you have no idea what they are talking about. This keeps you connected to their hobbies and interests. You will also quickly notice any sudden mood or behavior changes that could signify a problem.

> **No Private Social Media.** They are NOT old enough for unsupervised media. Social media has made it easy for children to heckle, harass and torment their target anywhere and anytime. It could be out of pure maliciousness, a dare, or for page views on an online video channel. In most cases neither the bully nor the bullied know how to reign in a bad situation. This can lower self esteem and lead up to serious problems like depression and serious eating disorders. Especially if the bullies are targeting their weight or appearance.

Another problem with unsupervised social media is the need for attention. Dangerous eating related stunts like the cinnamon challenge, the cotton ball diet and bleach in foods are all byproducts of such attention getting behavior.

Limit screen time, including phones if they absolutely must have them. Keep in mind their phones, game consoles and tablets can all pick up on other people's Wi-Fi networks.

Safety Tip: There are many great apps that will 'lock' the internet and apps on these devices until you are ready to allocate screen time.

> **Know The Signs**. Talk to your Pediatrician or family doctor about the signs of eating disorders like anorexia (starving oneself) and bulimia (eating vast amounts, and throwing it up

moments later). The sooner they are caught, the easier they are to treat. **A free detailed written and audio copy of the signs, dangers and treatments can be found at kidshealth.org**.

➢ **Intervene**. If you suspect your child has an eating disorder, contact a child nutritionist to get detailed information of the current ways to confirm, confront, and treat the problem. Make sure to keep in touch. An eating disorder is not like a weekend fad. It ingrains itself into their behavior patterns and belief system. It will likely take counseling and expert intervention to root out the source and repair the damage.

➢ **Learn About Community Service Opportunities**. There are farms, community centers, hospitals, and libraries that let families and youth volunteer. Giving back to the community is a great way to bond with your growing child. It can also give them a fresh boost in their self-esteem when they make a difference in someone's life.

➢ **Emphasize Healthy Eating Is For Life, Not Weight**. This is especially important if the healthier lifestyle is new to your child. Children can easily think the loss of sweets and hamburgers is because they are 'fat,' especially if they have been teased about their appearances. Place an emphasis on the long term goals: energy, mental clarity, and specific healthy details like strong hearts and stable blood sugar.

Helpful Note: Do not simply go with 'you will be healthier.' Many health awareness classes and guest speeches attribute good health with a child's weight. While a healthy weight is an important factor, **the actual end goal is to improve the quality of their life**.

The grade-school years are full of change and development. However, the key to mastering the chaos is mindfulness. As long as you stay engaged with your child's life, you will have the knowledge you need to keep them on a healthy diet. You will also be able to recognize the early warning signs of various troubles like peer pressure and eating disorders. With an open mind and a little planning, you can help your children navigate through these challenging years.

Chapter 6: Conclusion

*The groundwork of all happiness is good health. – **Leah Hunt***

A habit of healthy eating is one of the best gifts that you can give your child. Good nutrition gives them the energy, physical stamina, and mental clarity to tackle the challenges they face in life. It is never too late to start a new healthy lifestyle. In fact, you can make a positive change as early as today! Simply switch out sugary drinks for water.

Life has a way of trying to take over and sabotage your healthy lifestyle. However, every situation has simple and practical solutions to keep the poor choices under control. You can make healthy versions of practically any food from scratch. You can purchase healthier foods and ingredients locally. You can change out food for a more productive reward system. You can even provide better choices at school or at a party.

In addition, you can teach your child how to make good eating choices. As they continue to grow and develop, the healthy choices you make will deeply impact their attitudes toward healthy living. Set them on their journey with all the right tools to get them to their goals.

Appendix 1: Food Allergy Journal example

Use to keep track of the foods you introduce, their ingredients, and effects to narrow down possible food allergies and intolerances.

Date:

Food Introduced: _____

Observations:

_____

_____

_____

Day 2:

_____

_____

_____

Day 3:

_____

_____

_____

Safety Note: If adverse reactions occur, stop feeding and see if symptoms clear up. If serious symptoms occur, consult pediatrician or an urgent care facility immediately.

Appendix 2: Sitter Guide

Meal:

Time:

Menu:

_____

_____

Directions: (Ex: In fridge, warm in microwave 3 mins and stir)

_____

_____

_____

Snacks/ Times:

_____

_____

Allergies: (and where medicines are kept)

_____

_____

In Case of Emergency, Call: _____

References

Altmann, Tanya Remer, MD, FAAP, and Beth Saltz, MPH, R.D. What to Feed Your Baby: A Pediatrician's Guide to the Eleven Essential Foods to Guarantee Veggie-loving, No-fuss, Healthy-eating Kids. NewYork: HarperOne, 2016. Print.

Ansel, Karen/ Gowdy, Thayer Allyson (PHT)/ Ferreira, Charity, MS, RD.*The Baby and Toddler Cookbook: Fresh, Homemade Foods for a Healthy Start*. N.p.: Simon & Schuster, 2011. Print.

Hassink, Sandra Gibson., ed. *A Parent's Guide to Childhood Obesity: A Road Map to Health*. Elk Grove Village, IL: American Academy of Pediatrics, 2006. Print.

Hoeker, Jay L., MD. "Infant and Toddler Health." *Infant Botulism: Can It Be Prevented?* Mayo Clinic, 4 June 2015. Web. 20 June 2016.

Mercola, Joseph, and Ben Lerner. *Generation XL: Raising Healthy, Intelligent Kids in a High-tech, Junk-food World*. Nashville, TN: Thomas Nelson, 2013. Print.

About The Author

Dr. Duc Vuong is an internationally renowned bariatric surgeon, who is the world's leading expert in education for the bariatric patient.

His intensive educational system has garnered attention from multiple institutions and medical societies. His passion in life is to fill the shortage of educational resources between patients and weight loss surgeons.

Although trained in Western medicine, he blends traditional Eastern teachings with the latest in science and technology. Dr. Vuong was featured in TLC's hit show, 900 Pound Man: Race Against Time, and is currently working on his own weekly television show.

Using Periscope and Facebook Live @DrDucVuong, you can chat with him Monday-Thursday at 6 pm MST.

Visit Dr. Duc Vuong on

www.UltimateGastricSleeve.com

to learn more.

Other Books by Dr. Duc Vuong

...available on Amazon.com

Meditate to Lose Weight: A Guide For A Slimmer Healthier You

Healthy Eating on a Budget: A How-To Guide

Healthy Green Smoothies: 50 Easy Recipes That Will Change Your Life

Big-Ass Salads: 31 Easy Recipes For Your Healthy Month

Weight Loss Surgery Success: Dr. V's A-Z Steps For Losing Weight And Gaining Enlightenment

The Ultimate Gastric Sleeve Success: A Practical Patient Guide

Lap-Band Struggles: Revisit. Rethink. Revise.

Duc-It-Up: 366 Tips To Improve Your Life

Leave Me a Review!

If you enjoyed this book or found it useful, please take a moment to leave a review on Amazon. I'm always interested in learning what you like, think and want. I read all the reviews personally.

Thank you for your support!

Manufactured by Amazon.ca
Bolton, ON

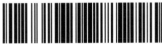

23756749R00035